Diana Rocha
Adilia Rafael
Sergio Sousa

Clinical Skin Challenges in Primary Health Care

Diana Rocha
Adilia Rafael
Sergio Sousa

Clinical Skin Challenges in Primary Health Care

The Portrait of Family Medicine

ScienciaScripts

Imprint
Any brand names and product names mentioned in this book are subject to trademark, brand or patent protection and are trademarks or registered trademarks of their respective holders. The use of brand names, product names, common names, trade names, product descriptions etc. even without a particular marking in this work is in no way to be construed to mean that such names may be regarded as unrestricted in respect of trademark and brand protection legislation and could thus be used by anyone.

Cover image: www.ingimage.com

This book is a translation from the original published under ISBN 978-613-9-61570-4.

Publisher:
Sciencia Scripts
is a trademark of
Dodo Books Indian Ocean Ltd. and OmniScriptum S.R.L publishing group

120 High Road, East Finchley, London, N2 9ED, United Kingdom
Str. Armeneasca 28/1, office 1, Chisinau MD-2012, Republic of Moldova, Europe
Printed at: see last page
ISBN: 978-620-7-86794-3

Table of contents:

Diana Rocha / Adília Rafael / Sérgio Sousa

CLINICAL CHALLENGES
CUTANEOUS
IN CARE
PRIMARY HEALTH CARE
CUTANEOUS CLINICAL CHALLENGES
IN PRIMARY HEALTH CARE

ACKNOWLEDGMENTS

To our families for their unconditional support at every stage of this long journey.

To our colleagues and friends for believing in the quality of our work.

GRATITUDE IS THE ONLY TREASURE OF THE HUMBLE

Shakespeare

AUTHORS

Diana Rocha

Master's Degree in Medicine from the Faculty of Medicine of the University of Lisbon. Family Medicine Intern at the Sete Caminhos Family Health Unit, ACES de Gondomar.

Adilia Rafael

Master's Degree in Medicine from the Faculty of Medicine of the University of Porto. Family Medicine Intern at the Sete Caminhos Family Health Unit, ACES de Gondomar.

Sérgio Sousa

Family Medicine Consultant at the Sete Caminhos Family Health Unit, ACES de Gondomar.

PREFACE

This four-chapter book reflects the reality of clinical practice in Primary Health Care. It shows the cross-cutting nature and diversity of the care provided by GPs and the immense need for them to be able to diagnose, treat and provide guidance, from the most common pathologies to very rare ones that are difficult to diagnose and whose delay in diagnosis could have a negative impact on the patient's clinical prognosis.

The topics covered in this book were inspired by four real clinical cases. The first deals with a rare and potentially fatal situation if an early diagnosis is not made; the second chapter portrays a very common pathology, pityriasis rosea; the remaining two chapters deal with situations that require high diagnostic suspicion in order to be treated accordingly.

They represent clinical situations which, despite their diversity, show the multiplicity of pathologies that the GP needs to bear in mind in his daily routine.

CHAPTER 1

STEVENS-JOHNSON SYNDROME IN PEDIATRICS: The IMPORTANCE OF EARLY DIAGNOSIS

DIANA ROCHA, ADÍLIA RAFAEL, SÉRGIO SOUSA

1.1. INTRODUCTION

Skin rashes are a common cause for consultation in primary health care.[1] Children are often the target of infectious conditions, not only because of their more vulnerable epidemiological context, but also because of the immaturity of their immune system. On the other hand, exanthematous diseases are frequent at this stage of life, making it extremely difficult for the doctor to diagnose the differential between dermatological diseases, since they share various symptoms and signs of presentation. The GP therefore needs to recognize not only the most common dermatological conditions, such as exanthematous diseases, allergic skin rashes and infectious diseases, but also diagnose more serious situations that are potentially fatal dermatological emergencies, such as Stevens-Johnson Syndrome (SJS).[2]

SJS was first described in 1922 in New York by two pediatricians (A.M. Stevens and F.C. Johnson) in two children with a generalized rash, fever, inflammation of the oral mucosa and purulent conjunctivitis.[3]

JSS is generally characterized by keratinocyte necrosis, which is clinically translated into epidermal detachment. In JSS, the percentage of detachment is less than 10% of the body surface.

1.2. EPIDEMIOLOGY

SJS is a rare pathology, with an annual incidence worldwide estimated at between 1.2 and 6 cases per million.4

The gender distribution is similar in children, while in adults it affects males more often.[5]

This syndrome is fatal in 5% of cases.

1.3. PHYSIOPATHOLOGY

The pathophysiological mechanism inherent in the SSJ spectrum is not clearly understood. The basic pathogenic phenomenon is thought to be a delayed hypersensitivity reaction.

There are individuals with a greater genetic predisposition to developing this pathology, namely those who are slow acetylators, those who are deficient in glutathione transferase (with an incidence of around 50% in the general population) and other enzymes responsible for metabolizing drugs.[6]

The cellular and molecular mechanisms inherent in this toxidermy have yet to be fully explained, although it is recognized that they are mediated by specific CD8+ cytotoxic T lymphocytes. CD8+ T cells recognize major histocompatibility complex I (MHC-I), modified by an antigen, and produce skin lesions characteristic of SJS.[6]

Activation of the membrane receptor Fas (present in the cell membrane of keratinocytes) by its ligand FasL, induces keratinocyte apoptosis through the activation of specific enzymes called caspases.

Recently, there has been a genetic association between certain alleles of the *major* histocompatibility complex HLA (*Human Leukocyte Antigen system*) and the development of severe adverse reactions to drugs, leading to SJS. Some of these associations relate to SJS induced by the combination of carbamazepine and the HLA-B*1502 allele in the Chinese population. On the other hand, the HLA-B*5801 allele has been associated with the development of SJS in Asian individuals medicated with allopurinol.[7]

1.4. ETIOLOGY

With regard to the etiologies that trigger JSS (Table 1), drugs are one of the most common causes, with B-lactams, anticonvulsants (carbamazepine, phenytoin, phenobarbital), sulphonamides, non-steroidal anti-inflammatory drugs (NSAIDs) and allopurinol being the most commonly identified. Antivirals can also be a cause of this syndrome.

Infectious conditions are the most common cause in children, where half of the patients had a recent episode of upper respiratory tract infection.

Neoplasms are also possible causes, although they are more common in adults.[8]

Despite the various etiologies, SJS is considered idiopathic in 25 to 50% of cases.[9,10,11]

Table 1: Drugs associated with SJS in children

PHARMACOLOGICAL GROUP	DRUGS
Antibiotics	Penicillins; Cephalosporins; Sulfonamides; Macrolides; Fluoroquinolones
Anticonvulsants	Carbamazepine, Lamotrigine, Phenobarbital, Phenytoin, Valproic acid
Others	NSAIDs; paracetamol, nimesulide; allopurinol; Chlormezanone, Nevirapine; homeopathic substances

Caption: NSAIDs - Non-steroidal anti-inflammatory drugs

1.5. CLINICAL MANIFESTATIONS

JSS is characterized by a delayed cutaneous hypersensitivity reaction that affects the skin and mucous membranes. It often presents with a prodromal phase characterized by general symptoms such as fever, malaise, myalgias and arthralgias. After these symptoms, a rash appears, usually not pruritic, which is characterized by erythematous macules with areas of confluence, which gradually turn violet, culminating in vesicles that confluence and easily rupture, giving rise to ulcerations and areas of necrosis of varying extent.

The pathognomonic lesion has a "target" appearance; Nikolsky's sign may also be present, which is characterized by the epidermis detaching when tangential digital pressure is exerted.[12,13]

The mucous membranes are affected in around 90% of cases, mainly the oral, ocular and genital mucous membranes.[14]

1.6. DIAGNOSIS

Since there is no specific diagnostic test, the diagnosis is clinical and requires a careful and complete clinical history, which questions the presence of the most frequent triggers.

Diagnostic confirmation requires a skin or mucosal biopsy.[15]

1.7. TREATMENT

When this syndrome is suspected, the primary treatment consists of the immediate elimination of the causative agent, when properly identified, as well as urgent referral to the hospital Emergency Department, since the prognosis becomes more favorable the earlier specialized care is started, and hospitalization in the Intensive Care Unit or burns unit may even be necessary.[16]

Support measures should be initiated with hydration, electrolyte replacement and a careful approach to the airway.

Eye damage requires observation by an ophthalmologist.

1.8. PROGNOSIS

Although extremely rare, given the mortality potential of this syndrome, the presence of certain factors seems to be associated with an increased risk of mortality in children with SJS, namely the presence of acute renal failure, septicemia and associated bacterial infections.[17]

On the other hand, the SCORTEN scale, preferably used in the adult population, could also be an important clinical tool for assessing the risk of mortality in these patients. It is based on the presence of certain risk factors (age, presence of a neoplasm, heart rate, degree of epidermal detachment, urea, glucose, bicarbonate), each of which is scored with a certain value, the sum of which predicts the risk of mortality.[3] (Table 2)

Table 2: SCORTEN Scale - Risk factors and respective mortality.

Risk factors	Score	SCORTEN	Fee Mortality
Age > 40 years	1	0-1	3,2%

Neoplasm	1	2	12.1%
Heart rate > 120bpm	1	3	35.8%
Epidermal detachment > 10%	1	4	58.3%
Urea > 28mg/dL	1	>5	90%
Glucose > 252mg/dL	1		
Serum bicarbonate < 20mg/dL	1		

1.9. CONCLUSION

JSS is a rare pathology, representing a dermatological emergency that is difficult to diagnose in the daily clinical practice of the GP. Therefore, whenever there are skin or mucous membrane lesions associated with taking drugs, viral infections, the presence of neoplastic conditions or simply lesions with some degree of diagnostic suspicion, urgent hospital referral should not be postponed with a view to early recognition and the start of appropriate treatment.

With tertiary prevention in mind, the GP should also be aware of the complications that can arise from SJS and which are associated with significant morbidity, such as synechiae, especially of the ocular and genital mucosa, and stenoses, especially of the gastrointestinal tract, secondary to skin re-epithelialization.

Ocular involvement can also translate into keratoconjunctivitis sicca, decreased visual acuity or even amaurosis[3] , situations which the GP should pay attention to with a view to early action (referral for periodic ophthalmic assessment, adequate ocular hydration with eye drops or saline solution, ophthalmic protection with sunglasses with ultraviolet protection).

CHAPTER 2

PITYRIASIS ROSEA: DIAGNOSIS and TREATMENT

SÉRGIO SOUSA

2.1. INTRODUCTION

Pityriasis rosea (PR) is a papulosquamous skin disorder, relatively common in clinical practice, first described by Robert Willan in 1798, but under different terminology. Subsequently, many names were assigned, such as Pityriasis circinata, Roseola annulata and Herpes tonsurans maculosus.

Typically, RP begins with the appearance of a larger erythematous scaly plaque on the trunk or neck, also known as a plaque, followed by the eruption of small multiple secondary erythematous and scaly lesions predominantly on the trunk and in the skin tension lines of the trunk and limbs, also known as Langer's Lines (Figure 1). [1,2]

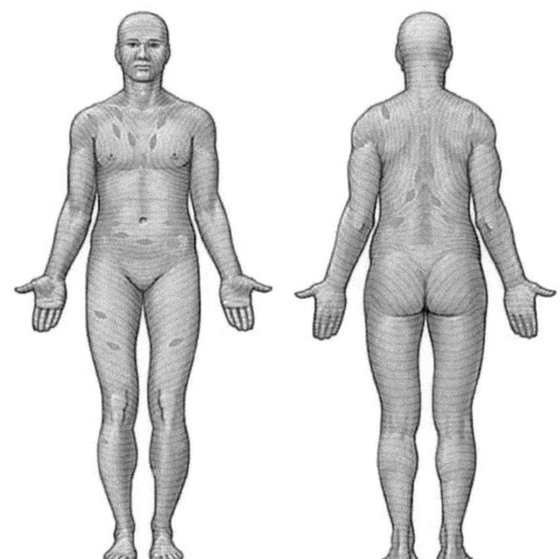

Figure 1 - Langer's lines. *Source: Villalon-Gomez JM. Pityriasis Rosea: Diagnosis and Treatment. Am Fam Physician. 2018 Jan 1;97(1):38-44.*

2.2. EPIDEMIOLOGY

The incidence of PR is 170 cases per 100,000 people per year, predominantly affecting people aged between 10 and 35 and affecting men and women equally. [2] The disease is self-limiting and in most cases the rash improves within two to eight weeks. A tendency towards familial *clustering* has been reported and prevalence is usually higher in winter. [2,3]

RP is a common disease in the GP's clinical practice and although diagnosis and treatment are simple in cases of classic presentation, diagnostic doubts often arise, especially in cases of atypical presentations.

2.3. ETIOLOGY

Numerous hypotheses have been put forward about the exact cause of RP, blaming both infectious agents such as viruses, bacteria and spirochetes, as well as non-infectious etiologies, specifically atopy or autoimmunity.

The epidemiology and clinical course of RP are suggestive of the etiological cause being an infectious agent.

The presence of familial *clustering* in some cases and the presence of a mother plaque (suggestive of a possible point of inoculation by the infectious agent), followed by the secondary eruption are also suggestive of an infectious etiology. An increase in CD4 lymphocytes and Langerhans cells in the dermis also points to a viral etiology[4] .

Recently, there has been an increase in evidence suggesting an important role for human herpes viruses 6 and 7 (HHV 6 and 7).[4]

HHV 6 typically affects children by the age of 2 and HHV 7 affects children by the age of 6. It is responsible for the sudden rash and it is thought that PR, which develops later, comes from a reactivation of these viruses[4,5] . However, the studies linking HHV 6 and 7 with RP are not very consistent and have certain biases that compromise the strength of the recommendations.

Despite this, these viruses are currently the most likely etiologic agents of RP and more studies are needed to establish a definitive link.

2.4. CLINICAL PRESENTATION

- **Classic**

The diagnosis of RP is based on clinical and physical examination. As mentioned above, typical RP begins with the appearance of a larger plaque in around 90% of cases.[3] The plaque is erythematous, slightly protruding and has scaly edges with a slight depression in the center (Figures 2 and 3). It can measure 3 or more cm in diameter and can be the only skin manifestation for approximately 2 weeks.

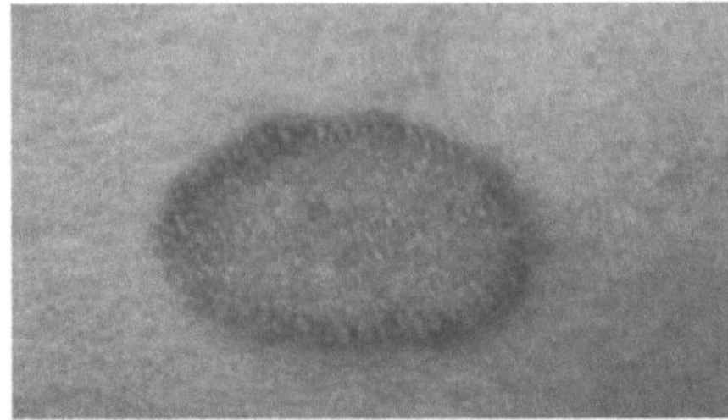

Figure 2: Pityriasis rosea mother plaque

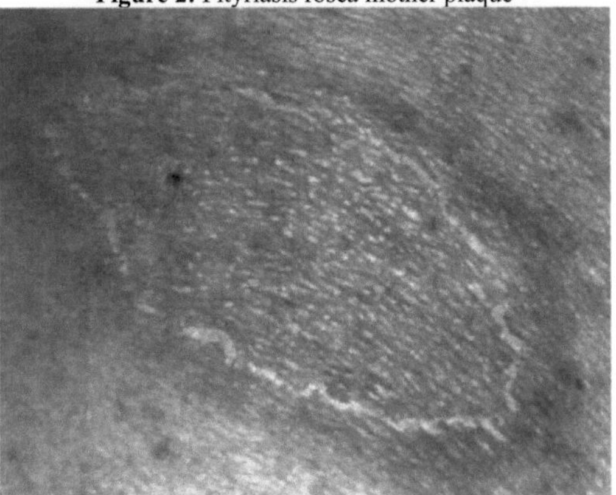

Figure 3: Pityriasis rosea mother plaque

Non-specific prodromal symptoms such as malaise, fatigue, nausea, headache, arthralgia, adenopathy, fever and odynophagia can be present before or during the rash in 69% of patients.

Generalized exanthema, also known as secondary eruption, presents on the trunk along Langer's lines (Figure 1) and can extend to the upper limbs and distal thigh regions. These lesions are smaller than the initial mother plaque and can continue to appear up to six weeks after the initial eruption (Figure 4).

The rash present in the dorsal region can acquire a "Christmas tree" pattern and the one developed in the anterior region of the chest, a "V" pattern.

The average duration of the rash is around 7 weeks, but it can last up to 12 weeks.[2,3]

Itching can occur in 50% of patients.[2]

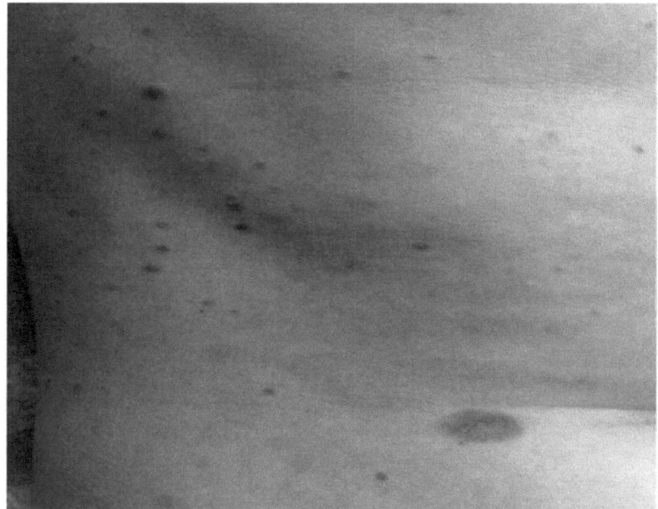
Figure 4 - Typical pityriasis rosea rash on the trunk with evidence of the mother plaque

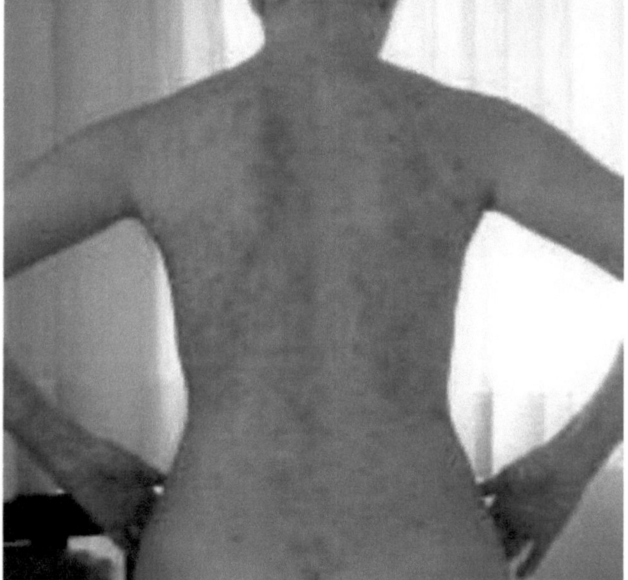
Figure 5: Pityriasis rosea on the dorsal region with Christmas tree distribution

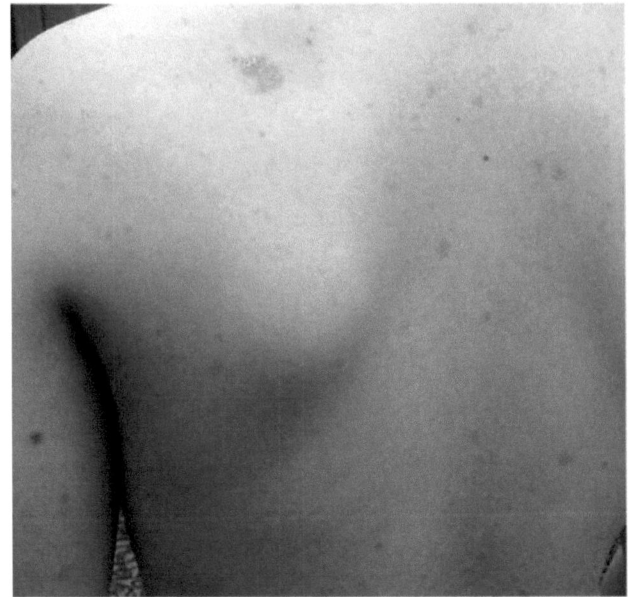

Figure 6: Generalized rash along Langer's lines

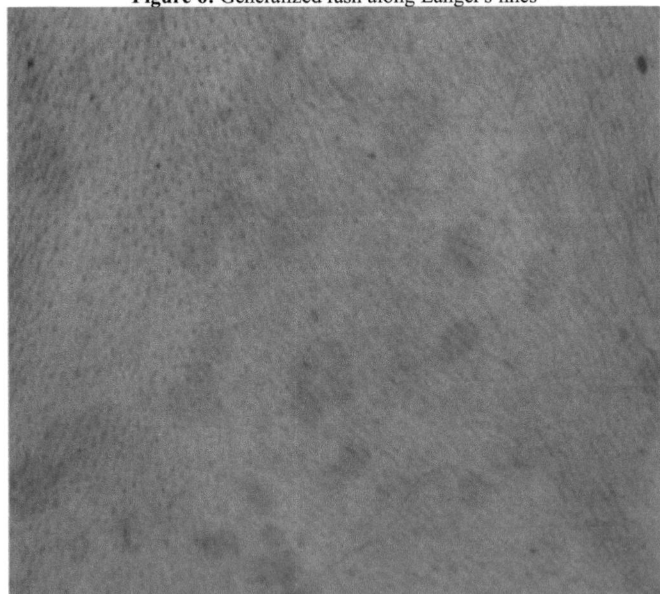

Figure 7: Typical lesions of Pityriasis rosea on the trunk

- **Atypical**

Atypical PR has a different distribution, as well as morphology, size and number of lesions.

The incidence of atypical PR is 20%.6

Most variants of PR are atypical in morphology but not in prognosis.

Some of the most common examples of atypical PR:

- Darier's pityriasis rosea gigantea - the patient has fewer lesions but they are larger.
- Pityriasis inversa - lesions predominantly involve the face, armpits and groin.
- Pityriasis Vidal - the rash is limited to the shoulders or the inguinal region.

2.5. APPEAL

The recurrence rate is low, between 1.8 and 3.7%, which suggests the development of immunity[2,5] .

Relapse typically occurs within 5 to 18 months of the initial episode.

When PR recurs, the mother plaque does not appear and the lesions are smaller and fewer in number. To date, the maximum number of recurrences described in the literature is five, and multiple recurrences of more than a few days are considered very rare. In these cases, it is suggested that certain clinical situations should be ruled out before diagnosing a recurrence of RP:

- VDRL test to rule out syphilis
- KOH to rule out dermatophytosis
- Consider biopsy if atypical lesions
- History of taking drugs that may be associated with a PR-type rash (Table 3).

Table 3: Drugs responsible for pityriasis rosea rash

Drugs responsible for pityriasis rosea rash	
ACEI*	**Vaccines**

NSAIDs**	**Barbiturates**
Omeprazole	**Bismuth**
Metronidazole	**Beta blockers**
Isotretinoin	**Penicillin**
****Angiotensin-converting enzyme* inhibitor**	
*****Non-steroidal* anti-inflammatory drugs**	

2.6. SPECIAL POPULATIONS

RP in children is similar to that in adults, but pruritus is more frequent in this population.

In the black population, the face is more frequently involved than in the general population. The eruption tends to be more pruritic and post-inflammatory hyperpigmentation is common.

Pregnant women are more susceptible to RP due to their altered immune status.

[3] This population deserves special attention as recently there have been reports of deleterious effects on pregnant women who develop PR and most doctors are unaware of this fact.[7] The miscarriage rate in one study was 57% in pregnant women who developed RP in the first 15 weeks of pregnancy. More studies are needed to establish a causal relationship between PR and adverse pregnancy outcomes and until then all pregnant women who contract PR should be closely monitored. In this group, treatment with acyclovir may even be considered.

2.7. DIFFERENTIAL DIAGNOSIS

The differential diagnosis of RP includes various pathologies (Table 4). If the diagnosis is dubious, skin biopsy may be indicated in very specific situations in order to clarify the diagnosis.

Table 4: Differential Diagnosis of Pityriasis Rosea

Differential Diagnosis	
Pathology	***Description***
***Lichen planus* pathology**	Violaceous papules measuring 1 to 10mm, well defined, typically present on the wrists, lumbar region, scalp, penis, mouth and leg. The lesions can be asymptomatic.
Nummular eczema	Small grouped vesicles of 4 to 5 cm, round or oval with distinct borders and an erythematous base, present on the back of the hands and legs, with intense itching.

Pityriasis rosea - drug-related rash	Similar presentation to PR, but lesions resolve after discontinuation of the causative drug.
Secondary Syphilis	Round or oval macules or papules, 0.5 to 1 cm in size, pink to reddish brown, scattered.
Tinea corporis	Protruding, scaling plaques of various sizes, with or without pustules or vesicles on the margins; lesions with relief of the margins and whitening of the center; itching.
Viral rash	Diffuse maculopapular erythema, with systemic findings of lymphadenopathy, hepatomegaly and splenomegaly.
Seborrheic dermatitis	Greyish-white or orange-red macules, papules or scaly plaques, with diffuse involvement of the scalp, worsening in winter, increased itching with sweating.

2.8. TREATMENT

The self-limiting nature of RP allows for an expectant attitude and only symptomatic treatment of pruritus in some patients where it is present and bothersome. Therefore, the use of oral antihistamines or topical or oral corticosteroids can be used according to current knowledge, taking into account the low potential for side effects of these treatments, however, they should be carried out for a short period of time.[2,9]

Other treatments have been tested, as will be discussed below; however, a *Cochrane* review did not show sufficiently strong evidence of their effectiveness:

- **Macrolides:** there is currently no evidence of the benefit of using these agents in the treatment of RP, and their efficacy is comparable to placebo.[10-12]
- **Antivirals:** the rational use of antivirals in the treatment of RP is due to the possible association between RP and HHV 6 and 7.
  Of the available studies, acyclovir has proved to be a reasonable option for the most symptomatic and severe cases of RP, although the results in the different studies are disparate. [13,14]
- **Phototherapy:** there are few studies evaluating the role of phototherapy in RP. Existing studies show a favorable response of symptoms and severity of RP to UV phototherapy, but more studies are needed before it can be inferred as a valid treatment option.[15-17]

2.9. CONCLUSION

Although much is known about PR, there are still some gray areas that need to be fully uncovered.

We conclude that the viral etiology is the most likely cause of RP and that antivirals may play an important role in the therapeutic approach to the most severe cases, and also in pregnant women.

All cases of suspected recurrence of RP should be properly studied before a real relapse is diagnosed, given the rarity of the situation, and special attention should be paid to pregnant women who develop RP, especially in the first trimester, given the association that has been seen with adverse effects on the ongoing pregnancy, requiring close monitoring.

CHAPTER 3

SQUAMOUS CELL CARCINOMA: A FREQUENT NEOPLASM WITH A PRESENTATION THAT IS SOMETIMES UNCOMMON

DIANA ROCHA

3.1. INTRODUCTION

In recent decades, there has been a significant increase in the incidence of cutaneous neoplasms in most European countries.

Skin cancer is the most common neoplasm in Caucasians.

Basal cell and squamous cell carcinomas are the most common, accounting for around 90% of all skin neoplasms.

It is crucially important for the GP to recognize cutaneous neoplasms early on, even when the form of presentation is not the most common, nor is the affected site the most frequent. It is known that the prognosis of these conditions is greatly influenced by early detection and rapid therapeutic guidance.

On the other hand, the role of the family doctor in preventing the disease should not be overlooked, reinforcing the primary prevention of the appearance of these lesions.

3.2. EPIDEMIOLOGY

Squamous cell carcinoma, also known as epidermoid carcinoma, accounts for around 20 to 30% of all skin cancers. Recent studies estimate an annual incidence of 70 new cases per 100,000 inhabitants for basal cell carcinoma and around 10 new cases per 100,000 inhabitants for squamous cell carcinoma.[1]

Squamous cell carcinoma is the second most common type of skin carcinoma in Caucasians and is more prevalent in the elderly.

Chronic sun exposure is one of the main risk factors for this pathology.

It occurs predominantly on chronically photo-exposed areas of the skin such as the face, trunk, ears and periauricular region, lips, forehead and scalp, and can also affect the upper and lower limbs. However, it can occur less frequently in areas protected from sun exposure, which requires a strong diagnostic suspicion.[2]

3.3. PHYSIOPATHOLOGY

The malignant transformation of normal epidermal keratinocytes is thought to be associated with the development of apoptotic resistance through the loss of functionality of the TP53 tumor suppressor gene. Mutations in this gene are detected in more than 90% of skin cancers diagnosed in the United States, as well as in the majority of precursor lesions of this neoplasm, suggesting that loss of TP53 function is an early event in the development of squamous cell carcinoma.

Ultraviolet radiation causes DNA damage through the creation of pyrimidine dimers, a process known to result in the genetic mutation of TP53. After subsequent exposure to ultraviolet radiation, keratinocytes undergo polyclonal proliferation, acquiring subsequent genetic alterations, ultimately leading to the development of squamous cell carcinoma.

Many other genetic alterations are thought to contribute to the pathogenesis of squamous cell carcinoma, including BCL2 and RAS mutations.

Similarly, alterations in intracellular signal transduction pathways, including the epidermal growth factor receptor (EGFR) and cyclooxygenase (COX), have been shown to play a relevant role in the pathogenesis of squamous cell carcinoma.[3]

3.4. RISK FACTORS

There are a number of well-identified risk factors for the development of squamous cell carcinoma, including: 8[4,5,6,7,]

- Over 50 years old
- Male
- Skin phototypes I and II
- Blue or green eyes
- Prolonged exposure to ultraviolet radiation (solar radiation, sunbeds)
- Exposure to chemical agents (arsenic, tar)
- Chronic immunosuppression
- HPV infection.

3.5. MANIFEST

Squamous cell carcinoma, which originates in the cells of the middle layers of the stratified sidewalk epithelium that forms the epidermis, often develops on pre-existing precancerous lesions. In the majority of situations, it appears on actinic keratoses, and can also originate from scars, ulcers and chronic fistulas, or in people who have had prolonged exposure to certain carcinogenic agents, such as tobacco, x-rays, arsenic, tar or derivatives.

On objective examination, the head and neck should be carefully assessed, as they are sites with a high incidence of this neoplasm (Figure 1).

The following characteristics of the injury should be taken into account:

- Location
- Contours
- Coloring
- Dimensions
- Texture
- Assess the existence of potential precursor lesions (crust, ulceration, actinic keratoses).

Patients with multiple actinic keratoses have an estimated 6-10% risk of developing skin cancer.[3,9]

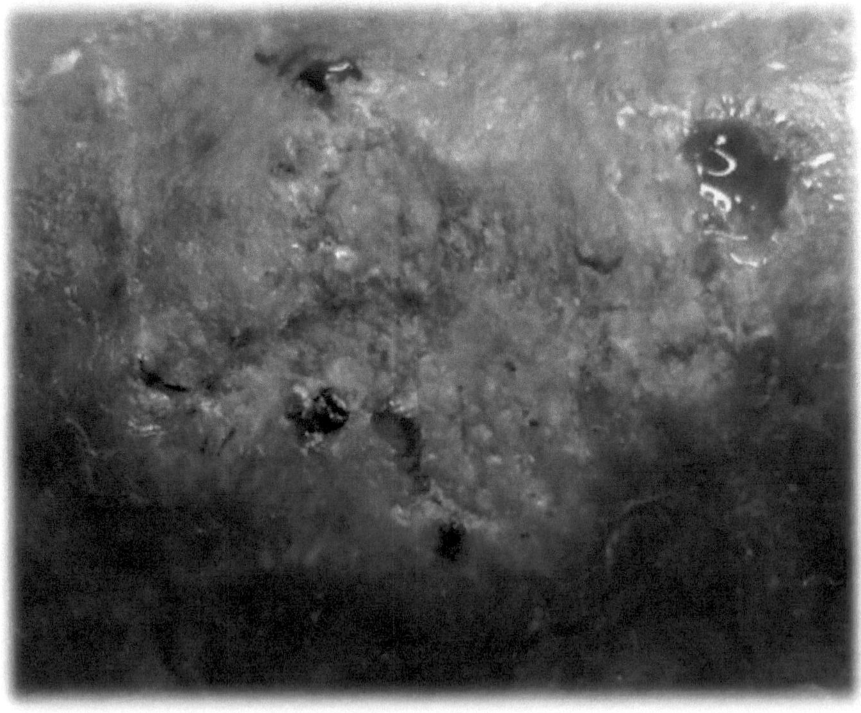

Figure 1: Squamous cell carcinoma of the leg

3.6. DIFFERENTIAL DIAGNOSIS

The differential diagnosis is extensive, however, we must take into account pathologies such as:

- Actinic keratosis
- Atypical fibroxanthoma
- Basal cell carcinoma
- Pyoderma gangrenosum
- Warts

3.7. DIAGNOSIS

The diagnosis of squamous cell carcinoma is based on a careful clinical history and a thorough physical examination.

A biopsy should be carried out on any lesion suspected of being a skin neoplasm, in order to rule out carcinoma or other dermal lesions.

3.8. TREATMENT

Treatment often involves surgery, with recession of the lesion in question, attempting to free margins from the lesion.

Some local treatments can be carried out in specific circumstances and taking into account each situation, such as curettage with electrocoagulation, cryosurgery, radiotherapy, *laser* application.

In addition to treatment, it is essential to maintain careful post-operative follow-up in order to detect tumor recurrences early (Figure 2).[4]

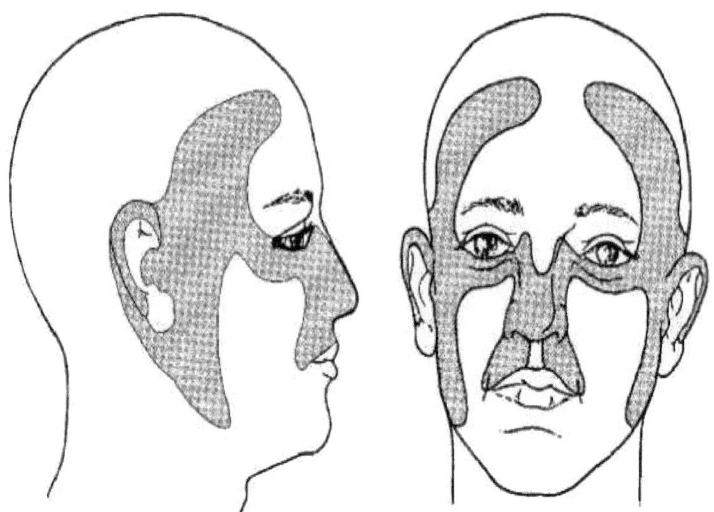

Figure 2: Regions of the face with the highest risk of recurrence of squamous cell carcinoma.
Source: Mohs Surgery Fundamentals and Techniques, Gross, K.G., Steinman, H.K., Rapini, R.P.; 1999, ed. Mosby; 12

3.9. PROGNOSIS

The prognosis for squamous cell carcinoma is favorable when detected early, with cure rates of over 95%.

Although squamous cell carcinoma is associated with a low mortality rate, it is associated with significant morbidity, especially when it involves the face. Most squamous cell carcinomas are located in the head and neck region, and the extensive excision required at an advanced stage of the disease can have serious physical and psychological repercussions. [1,2]

3.10. PREVENTION

Given the central role that ultraviolet radiation plays in the pathogenesis of squamous cell carcinoma, we can conclude that sun exposure precautions are of crucial importance in the prevention of squamous cell carcinoma. Furthermore, the treatment of precancerous lesions and carcinoma *in situ* can prevent the future development of invasive lesions with the potential to metastasize.

CHAPTER 4

PSORIASIS *GUTTATA*: A DERMATOSIS IN DROPS

ADILIA RAFAEL

4.1. INTRODUCTION

Psoriasis is one of the most common dermatoses in dermatology and is a frequent reason for seeking medical care, particularly in Primary Health Care (PHC). This inflammatory and chronic skin disease is recurrent and disabling, with a significant impact on patients' quality of life.

People with psoriasis can have different forms of the disease, ranging from plaque psoriasis (the most common) to erythrodermic, pustular, nail or *guttate psoriasis*. All of these represent different manifestations of the same disease, but in this chapter, the authors intend to focus on *guttate* psoriasis, precisely because it is one of the least common and with the fewest published studies.

4.2. EPIDEMIOLOGY

Guttate psoriasis (synonymous with guttate or punctate) is a rare entity, accounting for less than 30% of all psoriasis cases, and is more common in children and adolescents. It occurs equally in both sexes and rarely affects adults over the age of 30.[1]

Martin *et al.*[2] followed up 15 patients and determined that there was an associated 33% risk of developing chronic psoriasis within 10 years of the first acute outbreak of *guttate* psoriasis. Considering the 95% confidence interval, [11.8%-61.6%], this is quite wide, given the small sample of patients.

4.3. PHYSIOPATHOLOGY

The pathophysiological basis of psoriasis in general is characterized by aberrant proliferation and differentiation of keratinocytes, development of new blood vessels and infiltration of T lymphocytes, dendritic cells, neutrophils and other elements belonging to innate immunity.[3] Of all the subgroups of psoriasis, the *guttate* form is the one mainly related to streptococcal infections, which result in an immune response from T *helper* 17 (Th17) lymphocytes.[4]

This dermatosis has a strong association with the HLA-Cw6 allele, a genetic component that predisposes to the immune reactions that result in psoriasis, and is considered by far the most powerful genetic marker for the disease (*PSORS1* gene on chromosome 6p). One study even suggests a highly significant reaction, since all patients with *guttate* psoriasis have this allele, in contrast to only 20% of the control group.[5]

Recently, Qian *et al.*[6] published a study in which they evaluated the effects of peptidoglycan in the presence of cathelicidin LL-37 (a small peptide made up of 37 amino acids) in 28 patients diagnosed with *guttate* psoriasis, as well as the function of monocytes *in* peripheral blood *in vitro*. Peptidoglycan is the main component of the cellular appearance of streptococci and an increasing number of cells containing this molecule have been identified in individuals with psoriasis. On the other hand, cathelicidin LL-37 is overexpressed in psoriasis and is a multifunctional modulator of innate immune response elements, including monocytes. In *guttate* psoriasis, monocytes are activated, particularly the CD14 and CD16 populations expressed on the cell surface, which is regularly triggered by streptococcal infections. In this study, it was found that the LL-37 peptide induces differentiated monocytes, guided by peptidoglycan, in immature dendritic cells, showing increased expression of CD1a, CD86 and HLA-DR markers, resulting in the induction of proliferation and polarization of Th17 lymphocytes. The authors concluded that the LL-37 peptide, in perfect synergy with peptidoglycan, directs the polarization and differentiation of monocytes towards a pro-inflammatory phenotype, playing a key role in the pathogenesis of *guttate* psoriasis.

Scientific evidence shows an association between psoriasis and atherogenic dyslipidemia in several observational and case-control studies, even after adjusting for confounding factors (age, gender, obesity).[7-9] As a rule, psoriatic patients have higher plasma concentrations of total cholesterol, VLDL, LDL, triglycerides and lipoprotein A. In addition, there are low serum concentrations of HDL and apolipoprotein B. This type of profile may have been present since the onset of the skin disease (less than a year), suggesting that this dyslipoproteinemia may be genetically determined rather than acquired. Such a profile has been observed in patients with diagnosed *guttate* psoriasis, to which is added a genetic polymorphism of apolipoprotein E, which is clearly associated with dyslipidemia.[10] Despite the proven existence of genetic studies linking these pathologies, the pathophysiological relationship between them has not yet been fully established, but may be related to the increased production of pro-inflammatory cytokines, mainly TNF-a, leptin and IL-.

6, which play a major role in regulating the levels of lipids, free fatty acids and cholesterol observed in patients with diagnosed psoriasis.[11-12]

4.4. ETIOLOGY

In genetically predisposed individuals, environmental factors are essential for the development of psoriasis in general. By definition, *guttate* psoriasis results from an immunological reaction secondary to infections, whether bacterial, viral or fungal, as well as the use of certain drugs. Most of the studies in the literature on this condition affirm these facts.[13-17]

The first description of a correlation between strep infection and psoriasis was made by the English dermatologist Winfield in 1916. Its most common etiology is to occur one to three weeks after a respiratory infection (pharyngitis or perianal infection) with group A B-hemolytic streptococcus. More rarely, this variant of psoriasis appears after a viral infection or vaccination. However, it may simply be a chronic condition and not be associated with any previous infection.[18]

4.5. CLINICAL MANIFESTATIONS

The first clinical manifestation of this condition is the appearance of a multitude of droplet-like lesions (Figures 1 and 2). This dermatosis is characterized by the sudden appearance of multiple erythematous, scaly, rounded papules, which can even be pearly, ranging in size from 1 to 10 mm. They can be generalized or distributed predominantly centripetally (trunk) and on the proximal extremities and rarely affect the face, sometimes accompanied by pruritus.[1]

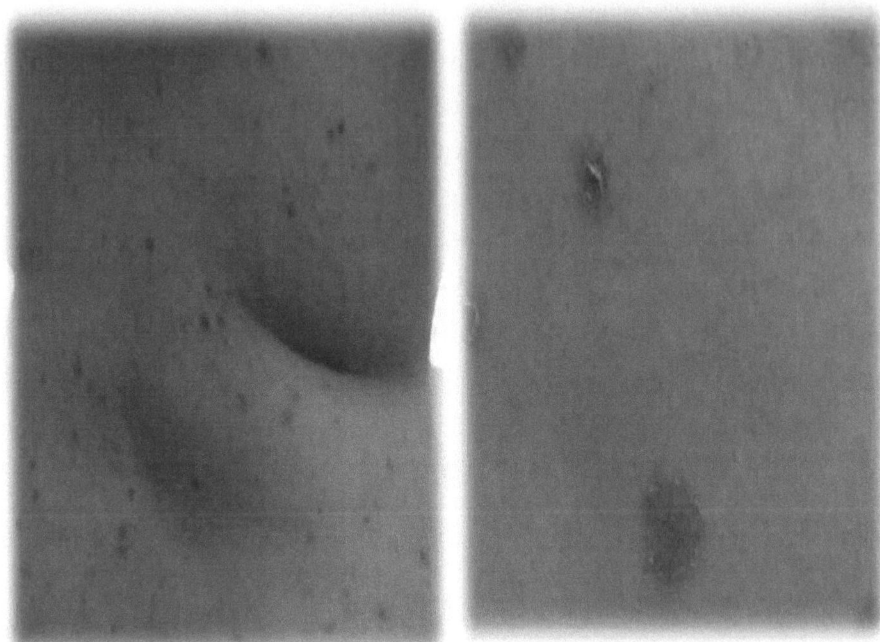

Figures 1 and 2: Erythematous and scaly lesions, predominantly located on the chest in a 31-year-old patient diagnosed with *guttate* psoriasis.

In the scientific literature, some cases of *guttate* psoriasis have been described, with some of the initial symptoms clashing, such as a history of fever, vomiting and abdominal pain, usually days/weeks before the rash appears.[19]

4.6. DIAGNOSIS

The diagnosis is often a suspicion, after excluding other pathologies with similar lesions (Table 1).

Because the main etiology is after a bacterial infection, they can appear during treatment with an antibiotic, and in some cases are diagnosed as an allergic reaction to the drug used. Amoxicillin is the first line of treatment for most bacterial infections; an allergic reaction to this drug usually appears eight to ten days after starting treatment, with the appearance of confluent macules and papules affecting a large area of the body. In the case of *guttate* psoriasis, these findings would be contradictory, given its predominantly centripetal location.[20]

Table 1: Differential diagnoses of guttate psoriasis.

PATHOLOGY	DIFFERENTIAL DIAGNOSIS				
	Incidence	**Localized**	**Peeled**	**Symptoms**	**Clinical aspect**
Psoriasis *guttata*	Children and young people	Centripetal and proximal ends	Little white flaking	Variable pruritus	Gouty, geographic lesions
Pityriasis rosea (*irritata)*	Young people and adults	Trunk, upper limbs and thighs (feet and wrists)	Thin, collared	Variable pruritus	Scaly plaques
Pityriasis lichenoides and varioliformis (acute form)	More common in children	Trunk and limbs	Absent	Fever and general symptoms precede in some cases	Drop-like" lesions slightly elevated, pinkish lesions that develop into crusts after necrosis
Pityriasis lichenoides / Chronic droplet parapsoriasis	More common in children	Trunk and limbs	Present	Absent	Similar to the acute form but does not develop into necrosis

Her body	More common in children	Trunk	Scales appear in some cases	Itching	Plaques with active edges and clear center
Leukemia *cutis*	Adults	Trunk (initially); widespread	Absent	Absent	Highly variable (papules, macules, nodules, plaques...)
Drug hypersensitivity reaction	Any age	Any location	Absent	Constitutional symptoms / anaphylaxis	Maculopapular rash and delayed urticaria
Secondary syphilis	Sexually active young people and adults	Symmetrical, face, palms, soles and anogenital region	Late, when there is no treatment	No itching	Macules, papules and adenopathies

In 2002, Eslick *et al.*[21] reported a case of a 27-year-old man who presented with several lesions confined to the trunk, erythematous, oval and accompanied by pruritus, initially diagnosed as pityriasis rosea. Due to the persistence and change in the clinical appearance of the lesions, the diagnosis was changed to psoriasis *guttata*. In this case, the final diagnosis was pityriasis rosea *irritata*, a rare variant of pityriasis, which in the later stages of development of the lesions, appear similar to *guttate* psoriasis; the atypical lesions on the patient's wrist and foot produced a diagnostic dilemma for the PHC doctor who initially observed him, and he turned to the Dermatology specialty to perform a biopsy of the lesions for a correct diagnosis.

Horlick *et al.*[22] also reported a case of a 62-year-old woman who was diagnosed with aleukemic cutaneous leukemia, a rare condition in which the patient had skin lesions containing leukemic cells before leukemia could be detected in the peripheral blood. In the case of the cutaneous manifestations of leukemia, they can be divided into non-specific lesions (leukemides) which do not contain leukemic cells and specific lesions (leukemia *cutis*). Their clinical presentation is quite variable and they can easily be confused with *guttate* psoriasis. In this case, the diagnosis was made by bone marrow aspiration which confirmed the result of myelomonocytic leukemia, four weeks after the appearance of the rash.

4.7. TREATMENT

Once it appears, it takes only a short time, usually weeks, for the problem to resolve, most of which does not require any treatment. However, in cases where there is an association with a previous streptococcal infection, the use of antibiotics is indicated, usually with a favorable response.[23]

Phototherapy has emerged as the first line of treatment, particularly in the moderate to severe form; the use of small beams of ultra violet light (311nm) has been shown to have good results, but is contraindicated in children. Options include narrowband, broadband or <) phototherapy. For patients who don't have easy access to phototherapy, controlled sun exposure is an option.[23]

Guttate psoriasis, particularly the mild form, responds well to topical corticosteroids, vitamin D analogues (calcipotriene), topical retinoids, calcineurin inhibitors and salicylic acid, which can be used as monotherapy or as an adjunct to phototherapy. Topicals are available in various forms, from ointments, creams, lotions, gels, *sprays,* foams and shampoos. Ointments are the most effective due to their lipophilic properties. If the first lines of therapy fail, it may be necessary to resort to systemic immunosuppressive treatments, which are normally used in the most severe cases of plaque psoriasis. Treatment with systemic corticosteroids is contraindicated due to the *rebound flare* phenomenon: temporarily there may be signs of improvement in the lesions, but when treatment is interrupted, the eruptions occur in a more extensive and severe form than the initial eruption, which can be fatal. [23]

Treatment with biological agents is not well defined for this type of psoriasis. At the moment, targeted biological therapy is reserved for cases of *guttate* psoriasis that evolve into chronic conditions, such as plaque psoriasis. [21]

Tonsillectomy may be recommended when there is a clear correlation between episodes of psoriasis and confirmed tonsillitis. However, more studies are needed to recommend this surgical procedure as routine.[24]

4.8. PROGNOSIS

As a rule, the clinical course is favorable, with spontaneous/self-limited resolution after a few days or a few weeks, often in children. However, it can reappear intermittently or persist and progress. In adults, it can reproduce the initial stage of another form of chronic psoriasis (plaque psoriasis), in around 30-70% of cases, even after a single episode of psoriasis 25 *guttata.*

CONCLUSION

Guttate psoriasis is a dermatological condition which, due to its uncommon nature, requires special attention from clinicians, particularly in the PHC setting, in order to recognize and treat it in good time. Considering the main etiology, *guttate* psoriasis should not be confused with hypersensitivity reactions to drugs, which can aggravate psoriasis if they are discontinued.

The existing scientific literature on this pathology is scarce and many of the publications refer to case reports from clinical practice. There is a need for more controlled studies with a larger population sample in order to better understand this entity.

BIBLIOGRAPHICAL REFERENCES

Papadopoulos AJ, Schwartz RA, Janniger CK. Chickenpox. Cutis. 2000 Jun;65(6):355-8.

Grimm L. 15 Rashes You Need to Know: Common Dermatologic Diagnoses. Medscape, Sep.
2015. Available at: http://reference.medscape.com/features/slideshow/skin-rashes

Das S. Stevens-Johnson Syndrome and Toxic Epidermal Necrolysis in Children. Indian Journal of Paediatric Dermatology, 2017; 9-14

French LE, Prins C. Toxic epidermal necrolysis. In: Bolognia JL, Jorizzo JL, Rapini RP, editors. Dermatology. Edinburgh: Mosby; 2003. p. 323-31.

Borchers AT, Lee JL, Naguwa SM et al. Stevens-Johnson syndrome and toxic epidermal necrolysis. Autoimmun Rev 2008;7:598- 605

Bulisani ACP, Sanches GD, Guimaraes HP et al. Stevens-Johnson Syndrome and Toxic Epidermal Necrolysis in Intensive Care Medicine. Rev Bras Ter Intensiva 2006;18(3):292-7

Chung WH, Hung SI. Genetic markers and danger signals in Stevens-Johnson Syndrome and Toxic Epidermal Necrolysis. Allergol Int 2010;59:325-332

Revuz J, Penso D, Roujeau JC et al. Toxic epidermal necrolysis. Clinical findings and prognosis

Hsu DY. Pediatric Stevens-Johnson Syndrome and Toxic Epidermal Necrolysis in the US. Journal of Dermatology Online. September 2016

ARS Norte, UPIP. Clinical Guidelines - Pediatric Ambulatory Care. September 2008. 56-57.

Colaço T, Espirito Santo M; Acyclovir in the treatment of varicella in pediatrics: an evidence-based review; RPMGF, 2009;25:424-8

Stulberg DL, Wolfrey J. Pityriasis rosea. Am Fam Physician. 2004; 69(1): 87-91

Chuh AA, Dofitas BL, Comisel GG, et al. Interventions for pityriasis rosea. Cochrane Database Syst Rev. 2007; (2): CD005068.

Drago F, Ciccarese G, Rebora A, Broccolo F, Parodi A. Pityriasis rosea: a comprehensive classification. Dermatology. 2016; 232(4): 431-437.

Rebora A, Drago F, Broccolo F. Pityriasis rosea and herpesviruses: facts and controversies. Clin Dermatol. 2010; 28(5): 497-501

Drago F, Ciccarese G, Rebora A, Parodi A. Relapsing pityriasis rosea. Dermatology. 2014; 229(4): 316-318.

González LM, Allen R, Janniger CK, Schwartz RA. Pityriasis rosea: An important papulosquamous disorder. Int J Dermatol 2005;44:757-64.

Drago F, Broccolo F, Zaccaria E, Malnati M, Cocuzza C, Lusso P, et al. Pregnancy outcome in patients with pityriasis rosea. J Am Acad Dermatol 2008;58 5 Suppl 1:S78-83

Drago F, Broccolo F, Javor S, Drago F, Rebora A, Parodi A. Evidence of human herpesvirus-6 and -7 reactivation in miscarrying women with pityriasis rosea. J Am Acad Dermatol 2014;71:198-9.Chuh A, Zawar V, Sciallis G, Kempf W. A position statement on the management of patients with pityriasis rosea. J Eur Acad Dermatol Venereol. 2016; 30(10): 1670-1681.

Amer A, Fischer H. Azithromycin does not cure pityriasis rosea. Pediatrics. 2006; 117(5): 1702-1705.

Pandhi D, Singal A, Verma P, Sharma R. The efficacy of azithromycin in pityriasis rosea: a randomized, doubleblind, placebo-controlled trial. Indian J Dermatol Venereol Leprol. 2014; 80(1): 36-40.

Ahmed N, Iftikhar N, Bashir U, Rizvi SD, Sheikh ZI, Manzur A. Efficacy of clarithromycin in pityriasis rosea. J Coll Physicians Surg Pak. 2014; 24(11): 802-805.

Drago F, Vecchio F, Rebora A. Use of high-dose acyclovir in pityriasis rosea. J Am Acad Dermatol. 2006; 54(1): 82-85.

Ganguly S. A randomized, double-blind, placebocontrolled study of efficacy of oral acyclovir in the treatment of pityriasis rosea. J Clin Diagn Res. 2014; 8(5): YC01-YC04

Leenutaphong V, Jiamton S. UVB phototherapy for pityriasis rosea: a bilateral comparison study. J Am Acad Dermatol. 1995; 33(6): 996-999.

Jairath V, Mohan M, Jindal N, et al. Narrowband UVB phototherapy in pityriasis rosea. Indian Dermatol Online J. 2015; 6(5): 326-329.

Lim SH, Kim SM, Oh BH, et al. Low-dose ultraviolet A1 phototherapy for treating pityriasis rosea. Ann Dermatol. 2009; 21(3): 230-236.

Associagao Portuguesa de Cancro Cutáneo; Basal cell and squamous cell carcinoma - available at www.apcancrocutaneo.pt.

Portuguese Society of Dermatology and Venereology; Skin Cancer - available at www.spdv.com.pt.

Najjar T. Cutaneous Squamous Cell Carcinoma. Feb 15, 2018. Medscape

Masini C, Fuchs PG, Gabrielli F, et al. Evidence for the association of human papillomavirus infection and cutaneous squamous cell carcinoma in immunocompetent individuals. *Arch Dermatol.* Jul 2003;139(7):890-4.

Wong SS, Tan KC, Goh CL. Cutaneous manifestations of chronic arsenicism: review of seventeen cases. *J Am Acad Dermatol.* Feb 1998;38(2 Pt 1):179-85.

Herman S, Rogers HD, Ratner D. Immunosuppression and squamous cell carcinoma: a focus on solid organ transplant recipients. *Skinmed.* Sep-Oct 2007;6(5):234-8.

Mehrany K, Weenig RH, Pittelkow MR, Roenigk RK, Otley CC. High recurrence rates of squamous cell carcinoma after Mohs' surgery in patients with chronic lymphocytic leukemia. *Dermatol Surg.* Jan 2005;31(1):38-42; discussion 42.

Nguyen P, Vin-Christian K, Ming ME, Berger T. Aggressive squamous cell carcinomas in persons infected with the human immunodeficiency virus. *Arch Dermatol.* Jun 2002;138(6):758-63.

Terzian L. Squamous Cell Carcinoma. IPELE Online Dermatology Book,2010

Motley R, Kersey P, Lawrence C. Multiprofessional guidelines for the management ofthe patient with primary cutaneous squamous cell carcinoma. *Br J Dermatol.*2002;146:18-25.

Fleming ID, Amonette R, Monaghan T, Fleming MD. Principles of management ofbasal and squamous cell carcinoma of the skin. *Cancer.* 1995;75(2):699-704.

Balow JE, Rosenthal AS: Glucocorticoid suppression of macrophage migration inhibitory factor. J Exp Med 137:1031, 1973

Martin BA, Chalmers RJG, Telfer NR. How great is the risk of further psoriasis following a single episode of acute guttate psoriasis. Arch Dermatol 1996; 132:717-718.

Nestle FO, Kaplan DH, Barker J. Psoriasis. N Engl J Med 2009; 361: 496-509.

Munz OH, Sela S, Baker BS, Griffiths CE, Powles AV, Fry L. Evidence for the presence of bacteria in the blood of psoriasis patients. Arch Dermatol Res 2010; 302: 495-498.

Zhang XJ, He PP, Wang ZX et al. Evidence for a major psoriasis susceptibility locus at 6p21 (PSORS1) and a novel candidate region at 4q31 by genome-wide scan in Chinese Hans. J Invest Dermatol 2002;119:1361-6.

Qian L, Chen W, Sun W, Li M, Zheng R, Qian Q et al. Antimicrobial peptide LL-37 along with peptidoglycan drive monocyte polarization toward CD14highCD16+ subset and may play a crucial role in the pathogenesis of psoriasis guttata. Am J Transl Res 2015;7(6):1081-1094.

Armstrong AW, Voyles SV, Armstrong EJ, Fuller EN, Rutledge JC. Angiogenesis and oxidative stress: common mechanisms linking psoriasis with atherosclerosis. J Dermatol Sci. 2011 Jul;63(1):1-9.

Schmieder A, Schaarschmidt ML, Umar N, Terris DD, Goebeler M, Goerdt S, et al. Comorbidities significantly impact patients' preferences for psoriasis treatments. J Am

Acad Dermatol. 2012 Sep;67(3):363-72.

Gerdes S, Mrowietz U. Impact of comorbidities on the management of psoriasis. Curr Probl Dermatol. 2009;38:21-36.

Gustafson B. Adipose tissue, inflammation and atherosclerosis. J Atheroscler Thromb. 2010 Apr 30;17(4):332-41.

Bays HE. "Sick fat," metabolic disease, and atherosclerosis. Am J Med. 2009 Jan;122(1 Suppl):S26-37.

Balci A, Balci DD, Yonden Z, Korkmaz I, Yenin JZ, Celik E, et al. Increased amount of visceral fat in patients with psoriasis contributes to metabolic syndrome. Dermatology. 2010;220(1):32-7.

Chalmers RJ, OÖSullivan T, Owen CM, et al. Interventions for guttate psoriasis. Cochrane Database Systematic Reviews 2000;2:CD001213.

Owen CM, Chalmers RJ, OÖSullivan T, et al. Antistreptococcal interventions for guttate and chronic and plaque psoriasis. Cochrane Database Systematic Reviews 2000;2:CD001976.

Tokura Y, Seo N, Oshima A, et al. Hyporesponsiveness of peripheral blood lymphocytes to streptococcal superantigens in patients with guttate psoriasis: evidence for systematic stimulation of T cells with superantigens released from focally infecting Streptococcus pyogenes. Arch Dermatol Res 1999;291: 382-389.

Telfer NR, Chalmers RJ, Whale K, et al. The role of streptococcal infection in the initiation of guttate psoriasis. Arch Dermatol 1992;128:39-42.

Leung DY, Travers JB, Giorno R, et al. Evidence for streptococcal superantigen-driven process in acute guttate psoriasis. J Clin Invest 1995;96: 2106-2012.

Mak RK, Hundhausen C, Nestle FO. Progress in understanding the immunopathogenesis of psoriasis. Actas Dermosifiliogr. 2009 Dec;100 Suppl 2:2-13.

Pinto M, Rios S, Guimaraes P, Oliveira T. Guttate psoriasis. Acta Pediatr Port 2012;43(6):273-4.

Saleh D, Tanner LS. Psoriasis, Guttate. StatPearls [Internet]. Treasure Island (FL): StatPearls Publishing; 2018 Feb 12.

Eslick GD. Atypical pityriasis rosea or psoriasis guttata? Early examination is the key to a correct diagnosis. International Journal of Dermatology 2002, 41, 788-791.

Berger BJ, Gross PR, Daniels RB, Lankton BB. Leukemia cutis masquerading as guttate psoriasis. Arch Dermatol 1973;108: 416-418.

Chalmers RJ, O'Sullivan T, Owen CM, Griffiths CE. Interventions for guttate psoriasis. Cochrane Database Syst Rev. 2000;(2):CD001213.

Chalmers RJ, O'Sullivan T, Owen CM, Griffiths CE. Interventions for guttate psoriasis. Cochrane Database Syst Rev. 2000;(2):CD001213.

Pinto GM, Filipe P. Best Practice Guidelines for the Treatment of Non-Pediatric Plaque Psoriasis with Biologics. Acta Med Port 2012 Mar-Apr;25(2):125-141.

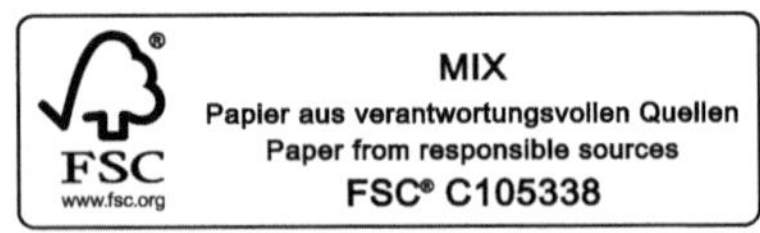

Printed by Books on Demand GmbH, Norderstedt / Germany